UPDATED

A YEAR OF **INSPIRATION, MOTIVATION,** AND **FOOD/FITNESS HACKS** WITH YOUR NUTRITION COACH

365 DAYS *of* HEALTHY LIVING

with
DAWN MCGEE

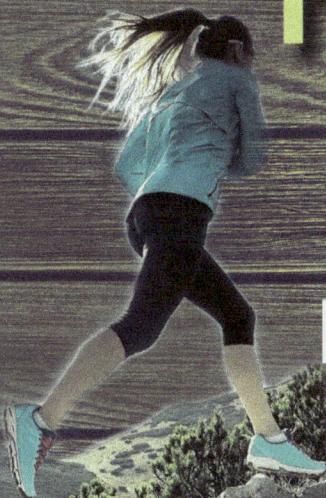

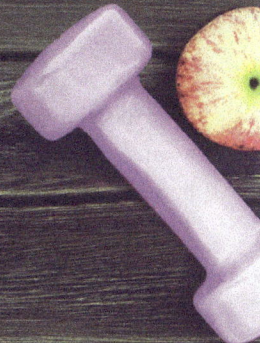

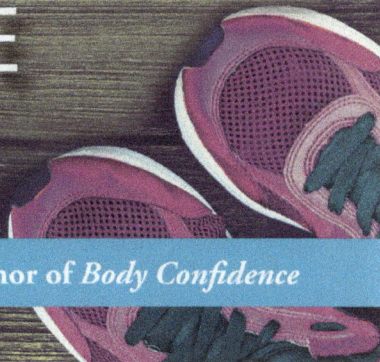

Foreword by Mark Macdonald, NYT best selling author of *Body Confidence*

Foreword

By Mark Macdonald

I've always felt there are special moments in life when you create a life-changing connection. For me, one of those moments was meeting Dawn McGee.

For the last few decades, my vision and mission has been to educate, empower and change the health of the world. But to accomplish a vision so big you must partner with powerful, like-minded individuals who share the same burning passion and commitment.

When I first met Dawn it was her quiet confidence that inspired me. There's an elegance to the way she speaks, coaches and writes about health that motivates you to immediately want to take action.

Dawn is a mom, wife, author, entrepreneur and world-renowned health professional and it's these life experiences that provide the calmness, knowledge and cutting edge strategies to help you win with your health, regardless of the busyness of life.

This is why I'm so excited for you to begin your health adventure with Dawn. Every word and page you read will be a positive step on the road to mastering your food, fitness and overall health.

As your adventure is about to begin, I would like to share with you the three best lessons I've learned from Dawn: Be Present, Stay Patient and Finish Strong

I know they sound so simple, but with every chapter of your life, new obstacles to great health pop up and of course, metabolisms evolve as we age. I've seen Dawn live these principles every day since first meeting her eight years ago, and I've watched her motivate and change so many people's lives, just leading by example.

The reality is you will have great days and not so great days, but if you implement Dawn's strategies and keep reminding yourself to be present, stay patient and finish strong, you will cross your health finish line like the champion you are!

Sending you the most massive hugs! Get ready, your health journey with Dawn starts now . . .

INTRODUCTION

I remember it just like it was yesterday. It was November of 2010, and I was just about ready to give in and buy larger clothes. You see, I had a delightful 6-year-old son, but I hadn't lost the "baby weight," and at that point, I didn't think that I could. And then I was introduced to the concept of blood sugar stabilization and eating PFC (Protein, Fat, and Carbs) ever 3 (every 3 hours), and it changed my life. I went from trying every fad diet on the market to never, ever needing to try another diet again because I was now in control over how I looked and how I felt.

Fast-forward to today. Welcome to *365 Days of Healthy Living*. I'm Dawn McGee, and I'll be your guide. Whether you are new to your healthy living journey or whether this is another tool in your toolbox of healthy living, I hope you find motivation, inspiration, and useful food and fitness hacks that you can use in your daily life. Let this book be a daily guide to keep you moving forward with your health goals.

Many of our daily pages have a foundation in the *Reclaim Your Life, One Bite at a Time*™ program I teach. I work with busy women to learn how to eat so they can feel healthier, and have more energy; all without being hungry, feeling deprived, or giving up their glass of wine with dinner. If you'd like to learn more and connect with our community, I invite you to join us in our free Facebook group, "Never Diet Again" (Facebook.com/Groups/NeverDiet).

If you have specific goals you're working towards (like losing weight, losing inches, decreasing body fat, or increasing energy), please write them in the space below. It's so important to break down your goals into small, simple, measurable chunks—which is what I teach you in my *Make This Your Year Goal-Setting Workshop*, which you can hop into at any time. I'm eager to help you on your healthy living journey.

Onward and upward!

Dawn McGee

Did you make any New Year's resolutions? Are there things you want to improve and change this year? The most commonly set (and broken) resolution is to lose weight. It's important to set yourself up for success with a solid support system and accountability partners. Share your goals online at facebook.com/DMNutritionCoach

RECHARGE

Is this going to be your year?
It can be! What small
changes can you make in
your life to move closer and
closer to your goals?

RECHARGE

Whether you took the Polar Plunge or stayed inside, I hope you kicked off your year with a clear and challenging workout plan. What changes are you planning on making to your workout routine this year? I'm planning on working my way back into a 5-day a week workout routine!

MOVE

Are you eating your rainbow?
Did you know that different
color foods have different
nutrients, antioxidants,
and health benefits? If you make
your plate as colorful as possible
(don't forget the protein and
healthy fats), you'll have a wider
variety of nutrients and flavors.
Enjoy!

EAT

They say that the best time to plant a tree is 20 years ago... and the second best time is today! Which is to say - it's never too late to make positive changes in your food habits. Remember: it's all about progress, not perfection!

RECHARGE

"There are two ways of spreading light; to be the candle or the mirror that reflects it."

-Edith Wharton

RECHARGE

Strong? Hell, yeah! What does strong mean to you? The strength to face another day? The strength to catch your kiddo when he leaps into your arms? The strength to bench press your weight? Whatever strong means to you, keep your workout progressions going until you reach your goal. It'll be worth it.

MOVE

Whether you're traveling or just hanging around town, it can be challenging to find on-plan food when you're on-the-go. Here are a couple of tips:

** Get a plain salad with dressing on the side and buy your protein separately - a hard-boiled egg with a couple of ounces of grilled chicken from a salad bar.

**If you're grabbing a pre-packaged meal, try for one that you can take apart so that you can eat the PFC (Protein, Fat and Carb) portions you want. Ask for double of the protein if there isn't enough for your portion. Many sandwich shops have apples and bananas by the cash register. Scout out the whole place before you decide what you're going to eat.

It is possible to stay on plan if you get caught without food on-hand. You can do it!

E A T

Life can be unpredictable, schedules can be overwhelming, and plans can change unexpectedly, leaving your workouts at the gym an improbable reality. Online workouts are a great option for those days when you know your gym workout won't happen.

MOVE

JANUARY 10

Be bold.
Do what the ordinary fear.

RECHARGE

Shoveling snow can be a good workout -- just be careful not to injure yourself. Lift with your legs instead of your back, and as with any workout, pace yourself. Trust me, the snow isn't going anywhere! If you shovel in intervals, you'll feel better. Remember: the best workout is one you can do again the next day!

MOVE

Busy week ahead? Meal prep for the week now. Like anything else, if you wait for the perfect time, it will never happen. Meal prepping will help you eat healthy and stay on plan without sacrificing your plan for the week.

Pro tip: Pre-cook your proteins and pre-cut your veggies so you can make a healthy meal quickly on a busy day.

EAT

JANUARY 13

There are times when life throws you curve balls. When that happens, don't lose your focus on your health. It'll help you better handle whatever life throws at you.

RECHARGE

WWW.DAWNMCGEE.GURU

JANUARY 14

How are those New Year's resolutions coming along? If you're like most people, your enthusiasm is starting to wane and you're wondering if it's really worth the effort. Think back to why you made these changes in the first place and what your success will mean to you. Community support is always helpful too.

RECHARGE

WWW.DAWNMCGEE.GURU

What changes have you made
to your workout routine?
How about adding more interval
training and HIIT to knock down
some of that extra body fat?

Haven't made any changes yet?
It's never too late to make tweaks.

MOVE

One of the best things about days off is that you can take the time to make a hot breakfast. Here's a classic: egg white omelet with veggies. Add in a handful of cashews, and it's a perfectly balanced breakfast!

What's your favorite?

EAT

Two weeks into the new year and it's time to track your progress. Measure yourself against your goals. Are you moving in the right direction? The great thing about tracking your results is that you have objective data and can make changes as needed.

Where there's a will, there's a way! You deserve to be healthy, too.

RECHARGE

"Believe you can and you're halfway there."

- Teddy Roosevelt

RECHARGE

What makes you happy? I'm in my happy place when my body is supporting me and I get to move. Exercise helps keep your mood positive and reminds you why you're working so hard to keep your food on plan. Enjoy!

MOVE

Have you ever found yourself staring into your refrigerator wondering what foods you could put together for a quick, healthy meal? Keeping a go-to list of your favorite clean foods can save you in a pinch.

If you forgot to meal plan for tonight's dinner, just pair a carb, protein, and fat for a quick, nutritious meal you'll feel great about.

E A T

Having a hard time kicking sugary snacks? Ask yourself why you're craving food you know is not good for you. If the answer is that you're hungry, grab fruit or veggies with some protein and healthy fat, like a hard-boiled egg or avocado. If you're not hungry for a healthy snack, chances are you're snacking out of boredom, so go for a walk and get re-energized!

EAT

Week three of the new year and you're probably starting to notice subtle shifts in your moods and self-confidence. These boosts come with taking steps to improve your health. It's never too late to get started.

RECHARGE

The weather can be unpredictable in the winter. Did it keep you from your workout? If it did, try some body weight exercises like push ups, squats, and crunches. Keeping a strong core will benefit you in many ways, both now and later in life.

MOVE

On plan dinners don't have to be boring! Swordfish sauteed in a non-stick pan with oregano and basil. Bell pepper rings with cherry tomatoes and mandarin oranges (with their juice) for sweetness. A handful of nuts for a healthy fat.

EAT

Let's face it. There's no silver bullet. Stop chasing the next best thing and get in touch with me to learn what actually works for your body.

RECHARGE

What do you wish for? More energy?
A smaller waistline?
Fewer health issues?
Whatever it is, eating clean brings
that wish a little closer to coming
true. What small change
will you commit to today?

E A T

Working out is key to staying happy, healthy, and focused. Today, I tried a new workout to stretch and tone, and I felt much better afterward. What do you do to keep variety and interest in your workouts?

MOVE

Favorite recipes can be made healthy. I transformed Caponata into an on plan meal. Eggplant, tomatoes, a little spinach seasoned with garlic, basil, and oregano, plus a smidge of olive oil as my fat. Paired with herbed chicked for dinner tonight. Paired with three boiled egg whites for lunch tomorrow.

E A T

What adventure does today hold for you? Make sure you pack PFC* snacks to take with you. Give your body the fuel it needs so you can live the life you want!

*Protein, Fat, and Carb every 3 hours

It's not always enough to know the information that can bring you success. You have to be willing to work for it. Why are you willing to put in the work?

RECHARGE

Sitting in an office chair or your car can take a toll on your core strength. Doing an exercise like the 'Superman' can increase core strength, improve posture, and get you out of your chair! Make a plan to get up and move or stretch a little every hour.

MOVE

WWW.DAWNMCGEE.GURU

Eating out can be challenging, but where there's a will, there's a way. We often go to Pizzeria Uno's for dinner (my son's favorite) and I order their salmon and steamed broccoli, both without salt or butter. I use a lemon wedge for flavor and have a wonderful dinner. Enjoy your dinners out and know that you CAN stay on plan!

E A T

"Be you, everyone else is taken."

-Oscar Wilde

RECHARGE

What would you give to feel completely free? There's no freedom in life like the one a healthy body can provide.

RECHARGE

Don't feel like you have enough time for a core workout every day? Try using an exercise ball instead of an office chair. It works your core and improves your posture, all while sitting at your desk!

MOVE

Hemp hearts are great to add to your repertoire! There are many ways to use them to pump up the "good for you" factor of your meals. Use them instead of bread crumbs to saute chicken breast.

Whether it's the doldrums of winter or other life stuff that's getting you down, it can be easy to forget to take care of yourself. Today, be a little more mindful of living intentionally, healthfully, and positively.

RECHARGE

What kind of culture are you creating? Does it nurture success?

RECHARGE

WWW.DAWNMCGEE.GURU

Finding the weather a little too cold to get outside for a workout? Turn your excuses into reasons. Find a corner of your house where you can do some simple exercises. Whether it's boxing, shadow boxing, jumping jacks, burpees, or planks, you can do a great workout in a small space. What workouts do you do at home?

MOVE

"Love yourself enough to live
a healthy lifestyle."

-Unknown

RECHARGE

Have your New Year's resolutions lost their zing? There's a great saying by Creighton Abrams about how to eat an elephant:
"one bite at a time"!

Reset your goals and bite off a little piece, something that you have confidence that you can achieve right now.

RECHARGE

FEBRUARY 11

Eat.

Transform.

Thrive.

RECHARGE

WWW.DAWNMCGEE.GURU

Karate teaches so many different skills. In addition to providing a great workout, they teach life lessons!

MOVE

Do you really know what you're putting into your body? Eating fresh, whole, and real food instead of processed junk food keeps our bodies healthy and our minds happy.

E A T

"Choose a job you love, and you will never have to work a day in your life."

- Confucius

Reduce stress and your overall health will improve.

RECHARGE

"Take care of your body.
It's the only place you
have to live."

- Jim Rohn

E A T

Be the boss of yourself.
Make time for your
workouts and enjoy them!

MOVE

"Eat crap, feel like crap.
Eat nothing, feel like doing nothing.
Eat well, feel well."

- Unknown

E A T

Seemingly impossible goals, like earning a black belt in karate, become possible when you break them down. It's the consistency of going to classes every week, the persistance of showing up even when you don't feel like it, the attitude that it can be done that makes it possible. Great life success lessons for all of us.

RECHARGE

"Every new day is another chance to change your life. "

-Unknown

RECHARGE

A great reminder for when you're feeling overwhelmed:
don't stress, real progress takes time. Grow from where you are, and you'll eventually get where you'd like to be.

What do you do to stay motivated when you're overwhelmed?

RECHARGE

"PFC Every 3" (protein, fat, and carb every three hours) keeps me full of energy and healthy all day long. We par-boiled some lasagna noodles, wrapped them around a scoop of filling, and baked them with sauce to make a yummy Stuffed Lasagna Noodle. Delicious!

E A T

There is an old saying that you can do something meaningful "full-time, part-time, or spare-time," but you can't do it "some-time." Whatever your goal is, set aside dedicated hours to do it. You can do anything in your spare time as long as you are persistent and consistent about it. What will you do with your spare time?

RECHARGE

"Life has no limitations except the ones you make."

- Les Brown

RECHARGE

When the weather isn't great, it's tough to get your bike out on the road. A kinetic trainer is a great way to get in some off-season riding. To round out your indoor workout, don't forget the foam rollers to smooth sore muscles, TRX + a kettlebell to strength train, and a mat for floor work.

EAT

"The best preparation
for tomorrow is doing
your best today. "

- H. Jackson Brown, Jr.

What do you do to prepare
yourself for tomorrow's success?
Meal prepping is a great way to
take steps towards success.

EAT

We make progress at the edge of our comfort zones! If you're feeling stuck or tired, challenge yourself to keep pushing; you'll see results and be grateful that you stuck with it. What will you do this week to expand your comfort zone?

MOVE

Some days, I don't want to work out. Sometimes, I want to sit on my deck with a book, a fluffy bagel with cream cheese and lox, and a mimosa. But I pour myself a little caffeine, make my eggs, and go to the gym. And I'm always glad I do.

Consistency and persistance will get you there. When you're faced with a choice, which do you choose? The easier path, or the one with the bigger rewards at the end?

MOVE

For a lot of people, working out is about losing weight. But what if we focused on non-scale victories, like getting stronger so we can lift our kids to the sky? Having more endurance so we can finish that 5k we've always wanted to try? Fitting into those jeans so we can look in the mirror and whistle at ourselves? Try it out today! Forget about the scale and focus on the reasons why.

RECHARGE

Sushi can be an excellent choice when you want to eat out but stay on plan! Be careful not to go overboard on sauces and seasonings, and enjoy a virtually guilt-free restaurant meal.

E A T

Food shopping and meal prep take time. One alternative is to use a shopping and meal prep service.

EAT

"Do what you can, with what you have, where you are."

- Theodore Roosevelt

RECHARGE

Are you off to the gym today?
Even when you don't want to go,
go anyway. 99% of the time,
you'll be happy you went.

MOVE

MARCH 5

What imprints in your life
have made you "you"?

Do they impact your
eating habits?

E A T

WWW.DAWNMCGEE.GURU

MARCH 6

Sometimes, you just need to take a deep breath and enjoy the day!

RECHARGE

Today is a new day. What small change in your perspective will make the difference between moving forward today and being stuck?

RECHARGE

Have you been eating clean and exercising, but you're still stuck on a plateau? Add in some HIIT to kick that plateau. More suggestions in the book, *Why Kids Make You Fat - And How to Get Your Body Back*, by Mark Macdonald.

MOVE

A healthy, gluten-free breakfast on the go! Using a muffin pan or 1c tempered glass cups:

1- Combine spinach, tomatoes, yellow bell peppers, and sunflower seeds.

2- Cover with three egg whites and bake for 40-45 minutes at 350°F.

EAT

Sometimes you just have to focus on what you can do and what you can control, and let the rest go. That will make all the difference in your day, week, and life.

RECHARGE

Sometimes you don't want to go to the gym or eat healthy foods. But exercise and eating healthy can be a boost for your mood. What do you do to get your day back on track if it seems to be drifting off?

MOVE

What's your favorite workout weather? When we have unseasonably warm weather, we take advantage of it and get out to the track to train a little bit. Whatever your workout plans, enjoy the day — enjoy the moments!

MOVE

MARCH 13

Ignite your metabolism, and learn how to eat for a lifetime. Starting the day with a healthy breakfast is important.

EAT

WWW.DAWNMCGEE.GURU

MARCH 14

Surround yourself with positive people and see how things change for you.

RECHARGE

WWW.DAWNMCGEE.GURU

Sometimes, you have to fight your way through the "no's" to get to the right "yes," especially when you are fighting with yourself about living a healthy lifestyle.

Keep fighting!

RECHARGE

When was the last time you replaced your sneakers? I shifted my workouts to kick it up a notch, and my feet were killing me! Well, I'm embarrassed to admit how long it had been since I replaced my sneakers. I got a new pair and felt much better! Make sure you get fitted somewhere knowledgeable.

MOVE

When you head out for the day and you're planning your MRFK (Mobile Readiness Food Kit), it doesn't have to be complicated with fancy cooking. Choose ready-to-go items and be on plan.
PFC every 3!*

*Protein, Fat, and Carb every 3 hours

EAT

MARCH 18

Practice positive thinking.
Catch people doing
things right. You'll be
pleasantly surprised
with how your life changes.

RECHARGE

WWW.DAWNMCGEE.GURU

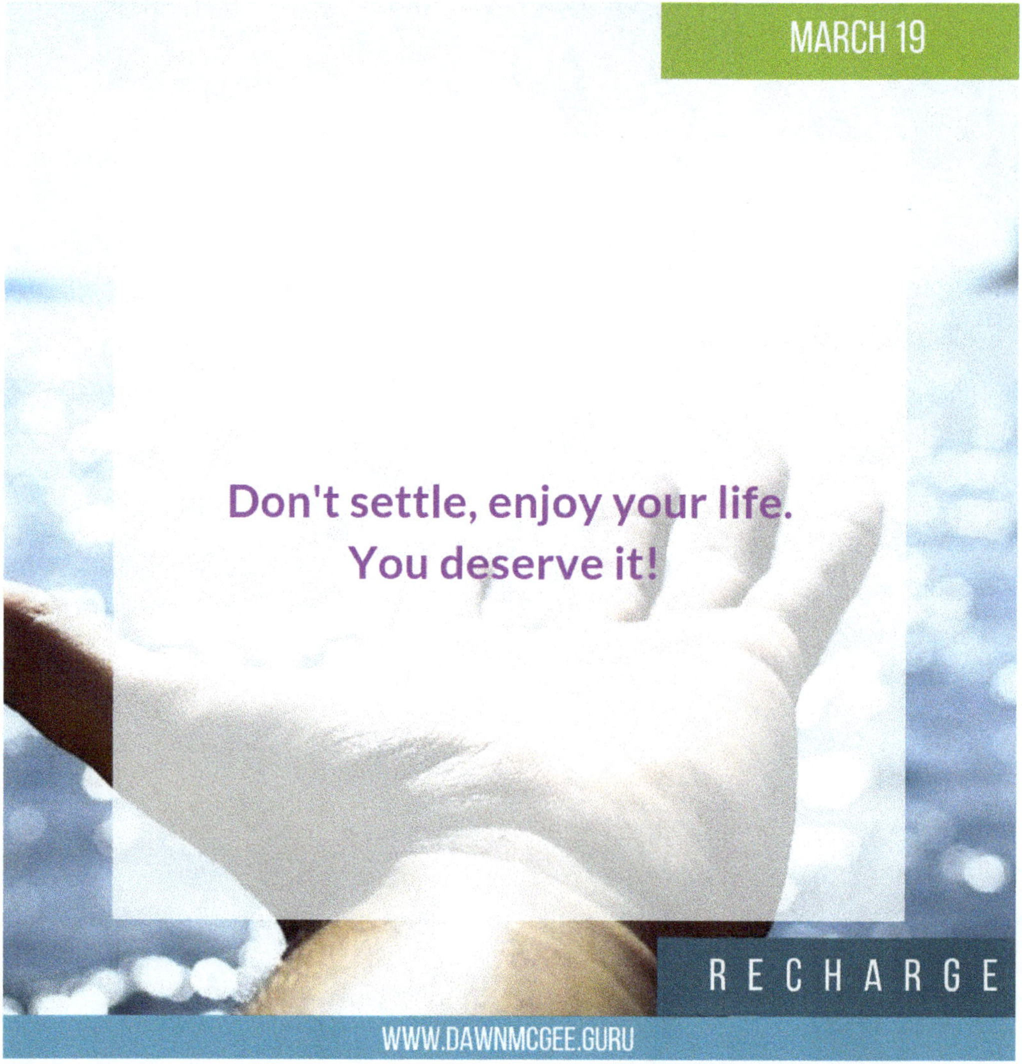
MARCH 19
Don't settle, enjoy your life.
You deserve it!
RECHARGE
WWW.DAWNMCGEE.GURU

Maybe you're focused on looking good in that bathing suit this summer, or maybe you just spent too much time snowed in this winter. Regardless of the reason, if you're getting back to the gym, go for it! Do it with both sensibility and intensity. Slow and steady wins the race, and also prevents injuries!

MOVE

What's for breakfast? Here's a great go-to meal. Egg white scramble with sweet yellow tomatoes and avocado. Seasoned with a little oregano. Kiwi on the side. Delicious, and balances my blood sugar.

EAT

Some days are tougher than others, that will always be true. Keep putting one foot in front of the other and you'll get through them. It will be worth it!

RECHARGE

"Keep going.
Everything you need
will come to you
at the perfect time."

- Unknown

RECHARGE

No one likes doing household chores. Period. But what if I told you you could knock out your chores and your daily cardio at the same time? Tidying up is a great way to score a solid workout without having to budget extra time for a jog or a trip to the gym. Turn up the music, cut loose, and dance to your favorite upbeat tunes. Engage your core muscles and stretch your hamstrings while bending over to pick up toys, shoes, or clutter. Do toe raises to tone your calves as you stretch to dust objects on high shelves or clean windows. The possibilities are endless!

MOVE

Want to add some fun to mealtimes? We played our own version of "Chopped." Our "basket ingredients" were: blue eggs, goat cheese, fresh pineapple, prosciutto, and fresh baguette. We made eggs, grilled baguette with goat cheese and prosciutto, and pineapple two ways (sauteed and as a base for the eggs for the grownups), garnished with strawberries. It was fun, and we all got to cook a healthy breakfast together. It's a great way to get your kids into the kitchen!

E A T

How you choose to look at things impacts everything in your life. Try choosing to see the glass as half full and see what a difference it makes.

RECHARGE

MARCH 27

Can you think of one thing that you can do today to get started towards your health goals? Just one. Remember, progress over perfection.

RECHARGE

WWW.DAWNMCGEE.GURU

Hey, we've all been there — life gets busy, and sometimes it's hard to find extra time and energy to devote to a real, sweat-breaking workout. Between parenting, work, and "life happens," your health often gets the short end of the stick, and it can seem impossible to get back on plan once you've formed bad habits around a busy schedule. Here are a few tips to get you on your feet and help you burn a few extra calories when hitting the gym isn't an option.

1. Just. Stand. Up. Really! Simply standing to do a rote activity (such as reading, making a phone call, or sending an email) can improve your health. Try a standing desk, or set an hourly reminder to stand up, stretch, and grab a fresh glass of water to give your body a break. Walk around while you're on the phone and get a jump on your 10,000 steps.

2. Move while you wait. Time spent waiting on a barista, traffic signal, or errant child who forgot to grab their homework can offer opportunities for lots of micro-workouts throughout the day. Pace, do calf raises, or knee lifts, or just move your feet from side to side to make the most of would-be wasted minutes.

3. Keep your core strong. It's the best anti-aging exercise. Whatever your job, whatever your schedule, it's easy to keep your abs engaged while you sit, stand, and walk. Imagine trying to touch your spine with your belly button and pull your stomach in accordingly, as often as possible. You won't get a six pack from this move, but this will improve core muscle tone when practiced with regularity.

MOVE

"Anyone can lose weight, the real challenge is keeping it off.

The three questions you must ask yourself when starting a food and fitness plan:

1. Is it based on science?
2. Can I do it for the rest of my life?
3. Would you let your kids do it?

Your answers to those questions will tell you everything."

- Mark Macdonald

EAT

I'm always happy when I get to attend in-person events and enjoy time with others who value health and wellness. Friends who can inspire you and hold you accountable are invaluable!

E A T

Every day we get a
new chance to start fresh.

It's essential for me to have a trainer to work with me, to hold me accountable and push me out of my comfort zone a little! How do you challenge yourself?

MOVE

Check out the book *Why Kids Make You Fat*! This is it — the way to regain control of your eating and your health. Enjoy a PFC* recipe from me featured in this book, too!

*Protein, Fat, Carb

EAT

The time of year for weird weather, fluctuating temperatures, and congested sinuses is upon us. Spring is great, but seasonal colds and allergies are not. Fortunately, nature supplies us with lots of foods that can help soothe sniffles, coughs, and sore throats. These are a few of our favorites:

Honey: You've probably tried tea and honey for a cold, but do you know why? Honey is naturally antibacterial, which means it helps fight off all the stuff that gets you sick in the first place. Choosing local honey can also help treat allergies by decreasing sensitivity to local pollens.

Licorice: Licorice is particularly great for couchs and sore throats. Suck on a licorice stick to reduce pain and nix annoying tickles in your airway.

Carrots: Cook them however you like; these soft, tasty veggies are loaded with immune boosting Vitamin A. They'll go down easy and boost your immune system while they're at it.

RECHARGE

"If something stands between you and your success, move it. Never be denied."

- Dwayne "The Rock" Johnson

RECHARGE

One of my favorite things to do on a day off is take a lovely walk with my son (and enjoy a delicious Dim Sum brunch). The sunny weather this time of year always puts me in a good mood, and a good workout helps keep me there. What is your favorite spring workout?

RECHARGE

Traveling can pose challenges for healthy eating, but staying on plan is possible. Choose an egg white omelet with spinach, mushrooms, and tomatoes along with a little Greek yogurt to keep a healthy gut. Keep your inner foodie happy and be confident that you are feeding your body well, too.

Pro Tip: If it's not on the menu, ask for what you want and they are usually happy to oblige!

E A T

Massage therapy is an ancient technique for soothing sore muscles and releasing stress. Excellent for addressing lots of different ailments, massage can be a great choice for people suffering from athletic injuries, anxiety and depression, pregnancy-related discomfort, or a whole slew of other issues. However, different massage techniques are intended to treat different problems, and when you're booking your first appointment, picking the right type for your body can be daunting. How does one decide?

Do your homework. Learn about popular massage methods and consider whether they apply to your situation. For example, Swedish Massage is a common, generally gentle and relaxing form of massage that releases tension from superficial muscle. Deep Tissue Massage, on the other hand, is a much more intense type of massage used to relieve chronically tight muscles, repetitive strain, postural problems, and other more severe issues. Figuring out what you want and what your body needs are the first steps to determining what type of massage is right for you.

Above all else, always be sure to discuss your body with your doctor or massage therapist to ensure that you safely receive treatment that fits your particular situation.

RECHARGE

Some days, it's easy;
some days, it's not. But if you keep
working at it, I bet you'll
be glad you did!

RECHARGE

How do you fit workout time into an already busy lifestyle?
Do you give up food prep time?
Do you give up sleep?
I hope not, as those are key components for your health as well. Maybe you do squats and lunges while doing food prep. It's time to get creative and get moving!

M O V E

If you're like me, breakfast is always a rushed affair (at least on workdays). It's always a temptation to grab a shake and skip the real food. But you can always squeeze in five minutes to make something, right? Try two eggs plus one egg white and some strawberries. Not the height of gourmet cooking, but yummy! It will fuel your body and brain so you're ready to rock your day! What's your go-to quickie breakfast?

EAT

"Eliminating the things you love is not wellness. Wellness feeds your soul and makes you feel good."

- Iman

Self-care is the cornerstone for everything in your life to work better. When you're healthier, you'll have more energy and clarity in everything that you do. This, in turn, will positively impact your relationships and your business. So take time to do the things that make you happy— consider it an investment with a guaranteed return.

RECHARGE

Life can throw a curve ball any time,
but if you keep moving forward,
even bit by bit, it won't
hold you back. Have a great day
and keep moving forward!

RECHARGE

Does your office job keep you sedentary? Put a reminder on your calendar or Fitbit to schedule movement breaks. Walk a lap (or two) around the building, grab a glass of water, run up and down a flight of stairs a few times. Once you get started, you may start a movement at work. Small changes make a significant impact over time.

MOVE

WWW.DAWNMCGEE.GURU

I love some extra *kick* on my meals, but the rest of my family doesn't, so I prepare theirs with minimal spice and then add some of my favorite Benito's Hot Sauce. No added salt or sugar, so I can use them knowing I'm putting something good and tasty into my body!

EAT

rseverance

My son gets a great workout at karate, but I'm guilty of spending too much time just watching instead of doing. Sometimes, all the moms get to participate with their kids. Mine informed me that he would not be taking it easy on me! What can you do with your kids instead of watching them? I bet they'll love it!

MOVE

"Age wrinkles the body. Quitting on dreams wrinkles the soul."

- Douglas Macarthur

I don't like wrinkles on my face or my soul! So I work hard at preventing both.

RECHARGE

Looks tough, doesn't it? If you practice every day, adding a few more seconds each time, you'll be able to hold the pose before you know it! Life is like that, too. Keep building your inner strength and working towards your dreams little by little. Before you know it, you'll be running across that finish line.

MOVE

I travel often so there is lots of restaurant food in my life. It's interesting how sensitive I've become to the amount of salt that most restaurants use in their food -- even when asked to prepare it without salt.

It is so satisfying to come home and make this meal, I just have to share it. It's a perfect balance of protein, fat and carbs - salmon steak seasoned with cayenne pepper and dill, steamed medium rare; spinach, grape tomatoes and baby portabellas sauteed in a non-stick pan with some spray. Mangia!

E A T

It's time to start thinking about longer days outside. Maybe you're eager to get your bike back on the road. Pack a PFC picnic and take the family with you! Picnics are a great way to spend quality family time and get some fresh air. What are some of your family's favorite healthy activities?

E A T

APRIL 20

What would you do if you knew you couldn't fail? Would you live your life differently?

RECHARGE

WWW.DAWNMCGEE.GURU

Don't let this happen to you!
Today was a day off from school, so we took our time and made a more leisurely breakfast. Egg white omelet with kale, spinach, avocado, tomatoes, and banana peppers. Sounds like the perfect recipe for a relaxing morning, right? Wrong! We waited too long to have breakfast and everyone's blood sugar was low—which makes for cranky, hungry people!

Keep your pacing, eat on plan, enjoy your day!

EAT

Healthy meals start with healthy ingredients. Shop fresh, organic spices whenever possible to give your body the head start it needs. Spices are key to beating mealtime boredom. You can have chicken 52 different ways with varying spice combinations.

E A T

APRIL 23

"What you believe,
you will achieve.
Why not believe
good things?"

- Mary Kay Ash

RECHARGE

Traveling? Busy? No time
or equipment for working out?
Here I am in Ottawa, squeezing
in some low impact cardio.
Stretching and body weight
exercises already done.
It'll boost my mood all day!
Where will you get your
workout today?

MOVE

Are your mornings rushed? No time for a healthy breakfast, or worse, no time for breakfast at all?! Try this perfectly PFC balanced bowl of cereal. Nature's Path Organic Flax Flakes with a handful of blueberries and protein shake mixed with 5 oz. of water instead of milk. Delicious, on plan, fabulous!

*Protein, Fat, Carb every 3 hours

EAT

Do you often feel like there just aren't enough hours in the day for you to take care of yourself? Even when your calendar is crazy, it's critical to prioritize physical activity and nutrition. Put an appointment on your calendar and treat it as if you were meeting with your most important client (which you are!). What are some of your favorite tricks for staying healthy on a schedule?

RECHARGE

There is no one giant step
that can make you healthy.
It's a lot of little steps.
Take your first little step towards
a better you today.

RECHARGE

Have you tried mug cakes?
You can have a lot of fun trying
out different variations. This one
is blueberry walnut. It takes
about one minute to
prep, two minutes to cook,
and voila! Healthy, delicious
breakfast in a cup.

EAT

Returning home from a trip sometimes turns out to be a longer process than planned. Fortunately, I had my shake packed for the flight, and I found yummy spinach, egg, and mushroom bao in the D.C. airport. It's so great to see how much airport food has improved in the last few years!

EAT

We all have those days.
Whatever your yesterday
was like, make tomorrow
better by choosing for it to
be better, even if it's just
a little bit better.

RECHARGE

MAY 1

Get inspired today by heading outdoors to celebrate the beauty of nature and soak up a little bit of Vitamin D.

RECHARGE

Do you worry about being bored with clean eating? Bring out your creativity! Try tilapia sauteed with spinach and tomato, spiced with dill and red pepper flakes. Delicious!

Every day is a new chance to succeed. What will you do today to get closer to your goal?

RECHARGE

Do your eating habits change when you have more time to cook and eat? Leisurely mornings are a great time to make a PFC* breakfast! Cooking and eating together gives us a chance to connect with each other. Sit down together for a tasty brunch while gearing up for the day ahead. It's going to be a great one!

*Protein, Fat, Carb

EAT

The first week of May is Teacher Appreciation week. Without the teachers in my life and my son's life, we wouldn't be as happy and successful as we are. I'm so grateful for all the wonderful teachers who give their all for our kids. If you know a great teacher, give them a hug and say thanks!

RECHARGE

Wouldn't it be great if we all had time to make fresh meals 5-6 times a day? Let's be realistic— most of us don't have the time and few of us have the desire to cook 5-6 times a day, every day. Pre-cooking some protein muffins, crustless quiches, or mini-meatloaves can be a lifesaver when you're on the run. Crustless quiches are my favorite way to avoid the dreaded breakfast skip. Try this recipe or adjust for your taste:

- In a 9x13 pan (spray lightly so it doesn't stick), layer fresh spinach and chopped veggies. I like chopped tomatoes, bell peppers, and onions.
- Lightly beat four whole eggs and eight egg whites.
- Season with rosemary, dill, pepper, or other spices.
- Pour the eggs over the veggies and bake at 350°F for 35-40 minutes or until the eggs are firm.
- This recipe yields four grab-n-go meals!

MAY 7

"Our bodies are our gardens;
our wills are our gardeners."

- William Shakespeare

RECHARGE

WWW.DAWNMCGEE.GURU

Too busy to cook lunch? Nah. Try this variation of Chicken Oreganata. The chicken was defrosted already, so prep took about five minutes and full cooking time about ten. Pound the chicken so it's thin and will cook faster, "bread" it with hemp hearts and a liberal sprinkle of oregano and parsley. Saute for just a few minutes on each side. While it's cooking, slice baby bell peppers and open a portion of mandarin oranges in juice. After the chicken is done, saute the peppers and oranges with some basil, letting the juice cook down a bit. Enjoy!

EAT

Does change terrify you?
Some people love change,
some don't. The only guarantee
in life is that things will change.
The question is this: how can
you re-frame your situation so
you can manage change in
small, bite-sized chunks?

RECHARGE

Many swear by body type dependent diets. The idea is simple: there are a handful of basic body types (endomorphs, ectomorpohs, and mesomorphs), and body type based diets focus on taking in more of certain types of foods depending on where you are likely to store weight.

Fortunately, you can check this off as a myth. Certainly, everyone is unique, and everyone's body will respond differently, but if you stick to your plan, you will have all the tools you need to succeed. Your basic plan is based on keeping your blood sugar stable and getting active so that your body can release stored fat. Have your first meal within an hour of waking up and eat every 3-4 hours until about an hour before bedtime. Each meal will consist of about 15-20 grams of protein, 15-20 grams of carbs, and 7-8 grams of fat for females (making each meal about 250-300 calories).

E A T

Do you know how many times Michael Jordan missed baskets? Many, many times. The most successful people are ones who just keep trying. What will you try today?

"The earth laughs with flowers."

- Ralph Waldo Emerson

RECHARGE

What's for dinner? Share a colorful, nutritious meal with your loved ones. Family dinner time has been shown to improve your child's perspective and reduce their susceptibility to peer-pressured bad habits. What is your go-to family meal? We love steak tips on the grill with grilled veggies or a big salad.

EAT

Every day, I make sure to get a good blend of colorful fruits for my antioxidants. How do you get your fruits and veggies every day?

EAT

This one is for my kiddo, who I'm super proud of! As a black-belt in karate, he has had many long days of testing, performing, and competing. Even on the days when he's nervous, he keeps going, knowing that he has prepared his best. What lessons can you take from this into your day?

RECHARGE

On the road again, with my favorite brekky- egg white omelet with veggies, a little salsa for color and some fruit.
The omelet station didn't list egg whites as an option, but they were happy to accommodate!

Change is tough. It's like being in a foreign country and not speaking the language. I coach people to embrace change and have patience as they learn new things.

Sometimes I travel for a couple of weeks at a time, and when I finally sit down to have breakfast at my house, I make my old standby: scrambled egg whites with veggies. Is it pretty? No! But it is comforting and delicious. Sometimes, amongst all the change, it's nice to curl up with a favorite, be comfortable, and just breathe for a few minutes. Then it's time to embrace the change again!

E A T

MAY 18

Don't forget to enjoy mindful eating today!

E A T

People are always watching
what you do. Do your best.

RECHARGE

Should I take lunch or buy lunch out?
I had some salmon already made.
I sliced up some cantaloupe and
honeydew, grabbed some fresh basil
from my plant outside, sprinkled
on some hemp hearts, and *voila*!
Under seven minutes and I had a
delicious, PFC* balanced lunch ready to
go. You can do it; I know you can.

*Protein, Fat, and Carb

EAT

"My own path towards wellness has been a long and dynamic one. It's taught me that healing from the inside out takes time and there can be great value in various sources of guidance."

- Carre Otis

Do you have changes you want to make in your nutrition and health habits? Plan a slow and steady course. It didn't take one day to get where you are, and it won't take one day to make positive changes.

RECHARGE

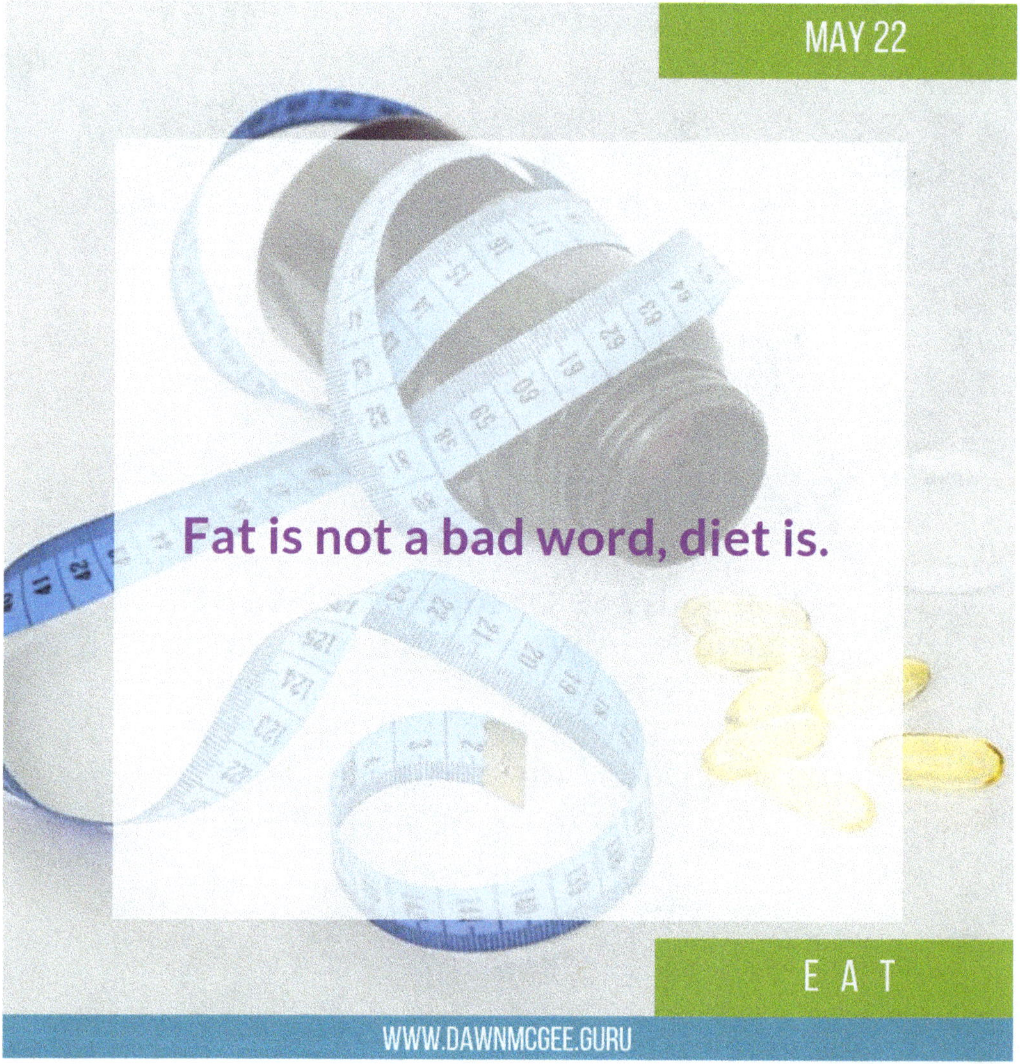
MAY 22
Fat is not a bad word, diet is.
EAT
WWW.DAWNMCGEE.GURU

Ready for a lunch break?
Don't skip this meal – you need
this fuel to keep your afternoon
chugging along. Add a grilled
chicken breast or a fish fillet to a
beautiful salad to make a
complete PFC meal. Farm fresh
veggies keep your
body and mind happy!

Life is best when lived
and enjoyed! What memories
did you make today?

RECHARGE

Making your own salad dressing is so much healthier than store-bought! Start with about 1/2 cup of your favorite healthy oil (sesame, peanut, walnut, avocado, or grapeseed). Whisk in 1/4 cup of acidic juice or vinegar (lemon or orange juice, champagne, or balsamic or rice vinegar), then sprinkle in flavor enhancers (garlic, shallots, honey, sriracha, tahini, herbs)... Be creative! Use a tablespoon of dressing on each serving of salad.

E A T

"He who has health has hope,
and he who has hope
has everything."

- Thomas Carlyle

RECHARGE

"Between stimulus and response there is a space. In that space is our power to choose a response. In our response lies our growth and our freedom."

- Victor Frankl

RECHARGE

Do you often have days where you're on the go all day? Put together an MRFK (Mobile Readiness Food Kit) with healthy snacks and water. When I'm hanging out at my son's karate tournament, I make sure I've got my MRFK to keep me fueled and my blood sugar stable. What's in your MRFK?

EAT

Start off right with a
healthy breakfast to keep
you energized all day long!

E A T

MAY 30

Another day of totally clean eating in the books and I feel great! What did you do today to improve your eating habits?

E A T

It's time to kick start your clean eating habits. Who's with me? Not only will you feel tons better, but you'll be part of a community of 10,000 enthusiastic people who are also working towards their health goals.
Come get your summer on!

RECHARGE

Vacation is right around
the corner. Don't lose your motivation.

Instead of blowing all your hard work by
eating junk food and lounging in the sand,
look for ways to make healthy choices on
vacation. Choose drinks with less sugar,
choose fruit over dessert, and take
advantage of an area's natural environment
to keep up with your workout. Activities
like paddle boarding, hiking, and bicycling
are excellent ways to enjoy your
destination and take care of your body
at the same time. Keep your eye on your
long-term goals and you'll be looking
hotter than ever when you return
home from your trip!

What are your favorite ways
to stay active on vacation?

RECHARGE

Warmer months bring an
abundance of fresh produce!
Raspberries make a great addition
to any meal because they're rich
in vitamins, antioxidants, and fiber.
You can add them to your shake
for a yummy fresh taste,
cook them down for a delicious
sauce for scallops, or add them
to your Greek yogurt.
Your imagination is the limit!

E A T

Our four-legged family members can be a great source of inspiration! Taking your pup for an extra-long walk is great for both of you and puts a fresh spin on your normal cardio routine. You can alternate intervals of fast and regular speeds for a great HIIT workout for both of you.

M O V E

Ten minutes! I walked into the kitchen and ten minutes later, I walked out with this dish! Chicken, shrimp, mini peppers, baby greens, tomatoes, and pine nuts sauteed in minced shallots and garlic. Yum!

E A T

Today, this is the entryway to my gym! June is a great time to enjoy 'Top 10' type days —sunny, light breeze, not too hot—so I went outside for a walk and enjoyed some fresh air. Although I enjoy my gym workouts, it's great to change it up a bit.

MOVE

Do you hate leftovers? I love them! I had a piece of salmon leftover from dinner and used it for lunch: warm tomato salad with salmon and fresh oregano. So simple, took me six minutes from start to finish. Fabulous meal, properly balanced to keep your blood sugar stable—and delicious!

EAT

How's your day going? Power through a tough day with a healthy snack. Fruit, nuts, and berries can give you that extra boost you're looking for. Add in some Greek yogurt (or your protein of choice) to blance out your meal and keep you fueled for the next few hours.

EAT

JUNE 8

Did you know June 8 is National Best Friend Day? Spend the day doing something fun and healthy with your friends!

RECHARGE

WWW.DAWNMCGEE.GURU

"What's for dinner?"
Chicken with spinach, quinoa, tomatoes, and garlic, paired with a Moroccan-style salad with cucumbers, tomatoes, red onions, a splash of peppery extra virgin olive oil, freshly squeezed lemon juice, red wine vinegar, and oregano.

E A T

**Never diet again!
Let's all learn how to eat
the foods we love,
and manage our healths and
weights. No deprivation,
no crazy diets.**

EAT

Do you get veggies from a local CSA? This egg scramble was 75% from mine — Farmer Dave's CSA. Tatsoi, fresh cilantro, fresh basil. Add a small handful of nuts, three egg whites, and veggies, and it's a PFC approved way to start your day. Enjoy!

EAT

Do you worry about how you're going to eat well while traveling? When prepping for a full day of travel, I spend 35 minutes in the morning (I prepare the chicken and fish ahead of time) to get my meals ready to be transportable for the day. Here's my menu:

Breakfast - Egg white omelet with spinach, tomatoes, avocado, hot banana peppers.
Mid-morning - Shake.
Lunch - Mahi and swordfish with tomatoes, baby bellas, sauteed onions, sunflower seeds.
Mid-afternoon - Shake.
Dinner - Chicken w gazpacho salad and sunflower seeds (in a Ziploc bag just in case it leaks).
Evening meal - Egg white and banana pancakes with peanut butter.

Since I'm traveling, I pre-make the pancakes. I'll wrap them in a paper towel and saran wrap. If I get delayed at all, I have an additional packet of shake mix, as well as some PFC balanced bars to help me out. All I need to do is buy some water once I'm through security and I won't have to worry about how I'm going to feed myself today. What are your favorite travel tips?

E AT

Are you counting down the
days to bathing suit season?
Let's dust off those healthy habits
and get back on plan.
Every journey starts with a single
step. Make today
the beginning of your journey
to a healthy lifestyle.

RECHARGE

Colorful meals = healthy bodies. Check out your local farmer's market for bright, healthy options! When you buy farm fresh food, you are getting a better nutritional value because it was ripened on the tree, not in a truck.

EAT

No time to meal prep? Think you can't eat a balanced meal without it? Think again! Even busy people can set themselves up for success. I don't always have time to prep, but I always have a piece of chicken in the freezer that I can defrost, slice, and sautee in about 15 minutes. While the chicken is cooking, I slice some strawberries and mini peppers, grab a handful of cashews, and voila! My PFC plate is ready to go. I feel pretty good about my Plan B skills, and I'll keep working on my meal prep skills.

E A T

"The world is changed by your example, not your opinion."

- Paulo Coelho

RECHARGE

Make a commitment
to yourself to eat a little
cleaner and work out a little
more intensely. You'll be
amazed at what a difference
that will make in just 8 weeks.

RECHARGE

Thank goodness for eggs! I always keep a bowl of hard boiled eggs in my fridge and when I need a quick, cold meal, I peel a few eggs, slice up some peppers, tomatoes, and avocado, season with oregano, wine vinegar, and in 10 minutes, I have a refreshing, delicious meal. If you're not a fan of eggs, you can swap in any other kind of protein (fish, chicken, etc.).

E A T

Life on the go!
I have my favorite cooler filled
with water, a shake, bars,
and extra shake mix just
in case I get stuck somewhere.
What's in your MRFK
so you can stay on plan?

E A T

Hoping to banish those last few pounds in a hurry? Be sure to combine high-quality protein foods with healthy fats and non-starchy carbs every three hours to ramp up your metabolism and keep your appetite sated.

EAT

JUNE 21

What are your nutrition goals
for this year? How is your
progress towards your goals?
That which is measured
can be improved.

RECHARGE

WWW.DAWNMCGEE.GURU

"Today, more than 95% of all chronic disease is caused by food choice, toxic food ingredients, nutritional deficiencies and lack of physical exercise."
- Mike Adams, the Health Ranger.

The foods we choose to eat affect both our short term and long term health. The lack of nutrition in fast foods and junk foods canpack on the pounds and leave your body in a state of chronic inflammation, which has a direct link to chronic illnesses.

Living healthily is an ongoing cycle. It impacts both your mental wellness and your physical wellness. Remember how good you felt last time you got outside in the sunshine and worked up a good sweat?

R E C H A R G E

Summer is just around the corner! Warmer weather brings opportunities for fun exercises like swimming, frisbee, and softball games. What is your favorite fun summer workout?

MOVE

Eggs get a bad rap, but they are one of nature's coolest foods. An excellent source of high quality protein, eggs also provide valuable nutrients like zinc, iron, and copper, not to mention lutein, which is great for your eyesight. My son likes his over easy; I like to scramble a few egg whites and one whole egg with some veggies for a refreshing, fresh breakfast. How do you eat your eggs?

EAT

On the road again. Having my PFC every 3 with a delicious and healthy breakfast. How do you stay on plan in a hotel?

EAT

Don't eat less — eat right.
Good nutrition is about how much
you're eating and what types
of food you're putting into your
body. Choose foods like leafy greens
and higher-fiber foods; they'll keep
you satisfied for longer, and they
won't spike your blood sugar as
starchy carbs will. Never skip meals;
your blood sugar will drop,
and you'll be more likely
to overindulge next time you eat.

E A T

Off-plan treats are great, but
do you really know what's
in your favorite coffee drink?
Flavored lattes, cappuccinos,
frappes, and similar beverages
often sneak in shocking
amounts of sugar and fat.
Don't be afraid to ask for nutritional
information before ordering at your
favorite coffee house, and pair it
with some lean protein so you
don't spike your blood sugar.

EAT

Nutrition doesn't have to be overwhelming! Connect with me in my Facebook group, Never Diet Again*, for tips on how you can start giving your body the nutrition it's craving.

*facebook.com/groups/NeverDiet

EAT

JUNE 29

Attitude is everything.
What you achieve is up to you.
What will you choose?

RECHARGE

WWW.DAWNMCGEE.GURU

It's Gazpacho season!
Gazpacho is my favorite cold soup.
There are tons of great recipes that
you can find - try a few different ones
to see what flavors appeal to you the
most. I like to add some hot sauce for a
little zing, and don't forget to add in
some protein to make it a PFC meal.
I usually add grilled shrimp. Enjoy!

EAT

Herbs help the flavors of food pop! Put a bed of fresh dill, oregano, and rosemary on your grill, then add salmon on top to infuse some delicious flavors into your fish.

EAT

Is now the right time
to change your eating habits?

Is it a struggle to fit in a healthy breakfast? Mornings can be tough— running around, trying to get everyone out of the house on time, and fueling yourself for your big day ahead! Try a little out of the box thinking. I made Chef Valerie Cogswell's Apple Turkey Sausages in a muffin pan and turned them into mini-loaves so I could grab one, add some fruit, and voila! Instant breakfast. It's delicious and the right balance of protein, fat, and carbs.

E A T

JULY 4

Happy Fourth of July!
How do you plan
to celebrate this great
country's birthday?

RECHARGE

WWW.DAWNMCGEE.GURU

Once upon a time, I would have just called this a meat and veggie casserole. Now, I call it gluten-free lasagna.

I had so much squash from my Farmer Dave's CSA that I didn't know what to do with it. We sliced them up, added some sauteed onions and scallions, put a layer of fresh tomato and basil in the middle, and slathered on the sauce. Looking forward to some great leftovers this week!

E A T

An intense workout can be very satisfying, but it's key that you don't overdo it! I've spent too much time in my doctor's office, wishing I hadn't twisted my knee and hoping that I had some non-surgical options. With summer sports, please take care to avoid injuries!

MOVE

For every success story, there are years of hard work behind it. When the USA Women's Soccer team won the World Cup for the 3rd time, there were years and years of practice and workouts that came first. Set your goals and then work the steps to get there, and you will.

RECHARGE

Every day is a new
chance to help someone
improve their life!

RECHARGE

Lunch on the road. Again. Fortunately, Japanese food has lots of wonderful options, especially if you go easy on the sauces. This salmon sashimi, octopus, scallop, and a spicy salmon/tuna roll (with very little rice), made for a great lunch and gave me the energy for the rest of my day!

E A T

What changes are you going to make in the coming days?

RECHARGE

Workout shoes? Hardly! But for a busy person, they'll suffice. Yes, I got in a walk. Yes, I did my strength training. But the day doesn't end there. Try to make your work shoes as comfy as possible so you can park further away from the door. Take the stairs as often as possible. Healthy movement is key to being a healthy you! Take your workouts wherever you go!

MOVE

As I explain to my son, life is not about competing with classmates. It's about improving yourself and being better than you were yesterday. How are you improving yourself today?

RECHARGE

Avoid the temptation of hotel breakfast buffets and order room service instead. It may be a splurge but you're worth it!

When you're looking for new workout ideas, pop into a convention to see the latest and greatest. IDEA World is a great place to learn about all the new fitness trends.

MOVE

"Knowing is not enough. We must apply. Willing is not enough. We must do."

- Bruce Lee

At IDEA World's Success Academy, Bruce Lee quotes are popular. It's no surprise, since he worked so hard to make himself successful. It's the kind of greatness we all have within ourselves. Set goals, work hard, and you'll see results!

RECHARGE

WWW.DAWNMCGEE.GURU

How important is fiber?
Very. Punching up fiber can
kickstart your weight loss and
help you stay satiated. Look
for foods with five or more
grams per serving to reap
the most benefits.

EAT

Mom always said,
"You are what you eat."
What are you eating
to be your best?

EAT

Would you like
to have more energy? Feel
good in your skinny jeans?
As we always say, "Great abs
are made in the kitchen".
Start today!

E A T

No matter how busy you get,
if your 'why' is meaningful,
you'll find a way to sneak
in some time to get moving
and get active. Your body will
thank you for it!

MOVE

Do you drink green tea?
It's high in antioxidants and
is said to help rev up
metabolism. Plus, it gives
you a caffeine boost without
being over the top.

EAT

Salads don't have to be boring! Check out this adaptation of a classic Nicoise salad: pan seared tuna, spinach/kale, grape tomatoes, baby bell peppers, garlic stuffed olives, and a little avocado. Top with your favorite extra virgin olive oil and balsamic vinegar, and it's a great meal for an early summer afternoon. It's a great PFC meal, but it's decadently delicious!

EAT

Many people have health and fitness goals that they don't quite know how to achieve. Or they might need a little extra motivation and accountability to get there. Working with a nutrition coach and a personal trainer can give you that accountability and motivation to get across the finish line.

MOVE

Get real! Eating whole foods and cooking at home as much as possible can make a huge difference in your overall nutrition. Keep a small garden (even apartment-renters can handle a dish of fresh herbs or a vertical garden in the window!) and cook with your loved ones to turn healthy meal prep from a chore into something you'll sincerely enjoy.

EAT

So, what's the plan? Establishing a nutrition routine can help prevent last minute stress from ruining your diet. Whether it's waking a half hour early for a run or focusing your grocery funds on fresh veggies, forming healthy habits is the way to stay on track.

EAT

For my family, warmer weather means fun in the great outdoors and delicious fresh fruit. A family bike ride or a walk to play Pokemon Go is always fun. What do you love most about summer?

MOVE

Salads don't have to be boring!
If you're choosing the same old
iceberg-lettuce-with-fat-free-
ranch pairing over and over again,
it's no wonder you feel burnt out.
Mix up your greens and add
interesting vegetables, fruits, and
nuts to your salad to keep things
interesting. Don't forget the
protein to make it a PFC meal!

E A T

Action-based goals are healthier and more sustainable than scale-centered goals. Instead of shooting to lose ten pounds, aim to shave thirty seconds off your mile time, increase your vegetable intake by one serving, or attend your favorite Zumba class every week for a month straight. Don't worry, your clothes will fit better and the scale will head downward, too.

MOVE

Rome wasn't built in a day, and neither are good habits. Incorporating healthy choices into already-busy lives can be overwhelming. If you honestly feel like overhauling your diet overnight just isn't possible for you, try staggering days at first. Committing to choosing salad for lunch four days out of the week or waking up early to exercise only on Monday, Wednesday, and Friday. That is a smaller, more manageable amount of change; you can always kick things up a notch later, when you feel more in control and empowered by the success you've already experienced.

RECHARGE

When I was young, I did not have good sun habits. I baked in the sun, used baby oil instead of sunscreen, and my skin used to show it until I found some great skincare products. Take care of your skin: it's the largest organ in your body, and it's the only one you've got!

RECHARGE

Avocado is a great source of healthy fat. You can add it to your salads with grilled chicken breast, or as an extra treat on a veggie burger.

E A T

"It's never too late to be what you might have been."

- George Eliot

Ever feel like you're too old, out of shape, and overweight to achieve the goals you used to have for yourself? After years of mistreating my body and recovering from serious injuries, I experienced my fair share of self-doubt on my wellness journey. I promise you, it's never too late to take that first step.

RECHARGE

"I'm too busy."
How many times have you said that? Now, I'm a crazy multi-tasker—I will stretch while wearing a Luminesce mask, while answering emails—but that may not be you. So whether you're in great shape or want to get into better shape, there's no time like the present! You may not have a beautiful lake like this to walk around, but wherever you are, pop on some comfy walking shoes and go on—get out for a walk. Your body and mind will thank you!

MOVE

Routines get boring. They also provide you with a structure for success. When my son goes away to overnight camp, I realize that I depend on our routines to be successful. Without them, I go out to dinner, have off-plan meals, and don't get up as early to workout. It's a good lesson for me: if I'm to be successful, it's up to me. This morning, a nice clean, PFC balanced breakfast - flax and oat flakes with blueberries and vanilla protein shake instead of milk. It took less than 5 minutes to make! What changes will you make today to be healthier?

E A T

Some will. Some won't.
What really matters is, will
you? I know you can do it.
I believe in you.

RECHARGE

AUGUST 4

Even the busiest people often take some time off in the summer. So you may lose some ground towards your goals. Don't worry! You did it once, you can do it again! And because you've done it before, you know that you can do it again. So get ready for that next "beginning," because you've got this nailed!

RECHARGE

AUGUST 5

I typically focus on your internal health, but let's not forget that our skin is super important to take care of too. Using sunscreen every day is key to keeping your skin protected. I finally found a moisturizer that has SPF30 in it, so my dermatologist is *finally* happy with me.

RECHARGE

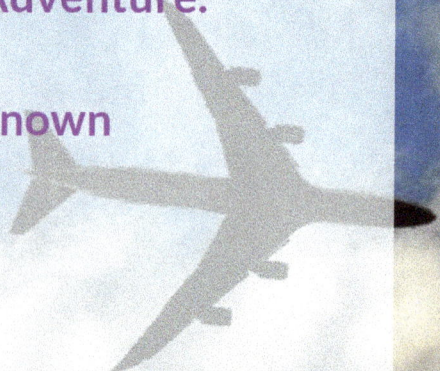

"Go, fly, roam. Travel.
Voyage. Explore. Journey.
Discover. Adventure."

- Unknown

RECHARGE

Staying active on vacation helps keep all that delicious vacation food from catching up with you! Biking, taking long walks, hiking, and watersports are all awesome ways to keep moving even when you're taking a break from reality.

MOVE

During lunch with a friend, I reflected on the fact that while I really enjoy clean, healthy, balanced meals, I don't love to cook. Since I also love to socialize, I'm thankful that places like Panera offer wonderful meals like this Mediterranean Chicken, Quinoa and Kale salad—delicious! Even though we may be out, or busy, or don't like to cook, it's still possible to eat well. Take a few extra minutes to read through menus, select a meal that has a good balance of protein, fat and carbs, and have the dressing on the side so you can add only what you need.

EAT

Do you subscribe to a local CSA for a farm share? It's so much fun to get surprised in your Farm Share veggie box and stretch your brain to figure out how best to use them.

E A T

Life is too short to be unhappy.
What small changes will
you make today so you
can smile more?

RECHARGE

Oh tennis ball—friend or foe? Yesterday, both. As I was silently cursing my trainer, I was using the tennis ball to roll out something in my glute that had gotten too tight and was restricting movement in my hip to the point of pain. Being able to release it was not fun, but it was a gift. Today, I'm better able to open up that hip and get back to doing real activities that I love, not just rehab. Sometimes we get so enthusiastic about our workouts and the expected results, we forget that stretching and other active release techniques are so key to keeping us healthy and moving forward. Don't forget to take care of your muscles so they can take care of you!

MOVE

What small changes can you make in your life so that you are not merely surviving, but thriving? Being more aware and grateful of what you have? Slowing down to enjoy the journey? Connecting more with the people in your life who truly matter to you? Pick a little something and have a great day!

RECHARGE

WWW.DAWNMCGEE.GURU

AUGUST 13

A stunning view of Mt. Mansfield in Vermont. If you're looking for a great workout while on vacation, hiking is a great option! You can go at your own pace, make it a cardio workout, or more of a strength training workout. However you do it, it's great to be outside, enjoying a change of scenery and some fresh air.

MOVE

WWW.DAWNMCGEE.GURU

On vacation in Vermont, we play volleyball all morning. Don't use extra activity as an excuse to eat off plan. Grilled chicken sandwich with Brie, roasted red peppers and mustard. Swap out potato salad for a green salad and don't eat the bread, and we're still on plan, with a delicious lunch!

E A T

Instead of arguing with people who think differently, think about how you can help educate them and raise them up. And also how you can educate yourself and be more open-minded. It is only when we help to grow others and ourselves that we will be truly successful.

RECHARGE

"My mission in life is not merely to survive, but to thrive; and to do so with some passion, some compassion, some humor, and some style."

- Maya Angelou

RECHARGE

AUGUST 17

What makes you
feel beautiful?

RECHARGE

WWW.DAWNMCGEE.GURU

Having the right mindset is the most important factor in success. What's the difference between most beach volleyball players and Kerri Walsh? She has a lot more belief in herself, and puts that to use on the court. Believe in yourself—go chase your dreams! What would you do if you knew you couldn't fail?

RECHARGE

Be real. Not perfect.
We all need this message sometimes, I'm sure. Be yourself. Always be working to improve yourself, but be yourself.

RECHARGE

When was the last time you tried something new? Summer is the perfect time for exciting activities like rope swinging, bike riding, and trail-blazing. Get outside today!

MOVE

It's not always easy to balance going out with eating well. What are your favorite restaurants with healthy (but still yummy) options?

I prefer outdoor walks.
Where is your favorite spot
for a little exercise?

MOVE

AUGUST 23

Summer is winding down!
How are you enjoying
the last few weeks
of sunshine and family time?

RECHARGE

AUGUST 24

"It always seems impossible until it's done."

- Nelson Mandela

RECHARGE

WWW.DAWNMCGEE.GURU

So you've heard that strength training is important, but do you know where to start? Research some great beginner's guides to strength training! When you gain strength and learn to sculpt your muscles, you'll end up with the body you've always wanted.

MOVE

AUGUST 26

What do you want most in life?

RECHARGE

WWW.DAWNMCGEE.GURU

AUGUST 27

Do your fitness habits match the work you put into your nutrition?

MOVE

WWW.DAWNMCGEE.GURU

"If your ship doesn't come in,
swim out to it."

- Jonathan Winters.

RECHARGE

We're all human. We all fall off plan. The question is, what do you do next? Don't be afraid to get back up and try again!

RECHARGE

Fresh blueberries, roasted chicken, baby arugula with balsamic and extra virgin olive oil. Yum! When you can be a little creative with your salads, it doesn't feel like the same old grilled chicken over and over again. What are your favorite salads?

E A T

We spend so much time working to keep our bodies looking young and healthy, but what about our minds? Did you know that eating healthy and exercising also stimulates mental health?

RECHARGE

For me, autumn is my time of renewal, resolutions, and planning. What will you do to make a measurable improvement in your health this fall?

RECHARGE

Here are all the ingredients to make a big batch of Gazpacho. What meals can you make in a big batch so that you have plenty of leftovers?

E A T

Gazpacho done!
With shrimp added for protein, it's a complete meal. It was a yummy gazpacho with layered flavors that packed a big nutritional punch.

EAT

Have you heard that sitting too much can make your butt bigger? A recent study at Tel Aviv University says that putting direct pressure on fat cells, like when you're sitting on your butt in your office chair, can cause fat cells to expand by up to 50%! More incentive to get up and get moving!

M O V E

A little while ago, I did a survey on how many people in my community take vitamins and which ones. I wasn't surprised to see responses all over the map. I work hard at getting my nutrients from food, but I know that I need help in some areas, so the AM & PM Essentials™ are my choice. I find that I sleep more deeply and have more consistency with my digestion. I love it! There are lots of great vitamins on the market. Find some that meet your needs and be consistent about taking them daily. In the long run, you'll be glad you did.

EAT

Some people make things happen. Some watch what happens. Others look around and wonder, "What happened?" Which one do you want to be?

RECHARGE

Fall is a great time to kickstart your fitness efforts. The kiddos are back at school, the weather is fabulous, and the outdoors are gorgeous. Take advantage of your increased motivation to recenter yourself and get back on track!

MOVE

Time for a seasonal clean eating detox? I usually start one in the fall to banish summer barbecue bloat. Here's a sample meal plan for you.

Breakfast: Start with a classic egg white scramble.

Mid-morning Meal: Zen Fuze

Lunch: Turkey with no salt and sugar-free mustard, kiwi, and cashews.

Mid-afternoon Meal: Shake #2.

Dinner: Seared tuna over salad.

Wrap up with a Zen Fuze vanilla shake blended with half a banana before bedtime.

It will make you aware of how much mindless munching you sometimes do. Time to banish that and up your water intake!

E A T

A few days into a super clean eating week is when my brain always starts to say, "Wouldn't a slice of pizza taste great right now?" This is the time to make sure my meal prep is solid. If I don't have a meal ready when it's time to eat, I'll invariably grab something off plan. The first few days are usually surprisingly easy, but planning for the tough days is crucial.

E A T

With just a hint of autumn in the air, it's a good time for self-reflection. What went well last year? What would you like to change in the coming year? How can you engineer your life so that you are living a life you truly love? What would you do if you really and truly believed that anything is possible? Spend some time each day in that place where anything is possible and watch your world open before you.

RECHARGE

This is the image of the NYC skyline that I grew up with. Many years ago today, the world looked on in horror as unspeakable acts of terror were committed and the Towers came down. Everyone was affected in some way.

As bad as that day was, we also saw a lot of good—people helping each other in truly amazing ways. So when we say Never Forget, let's remember that we saw the best in people as well that day, and keep that spark alive. What can you do today to put a smile on someone else's face?

RECHARGE

When you're looking to make
a change—any change, and
particularly with nutrition—you
need to let go of any past
successes or failures. Here
and now, you can do this.
I believe in you.

RECHARGE

Busy? Traveling? Can't work out? Nonsense. Look for this sign or one similar and have confidence that you are in a hotel where you can stay healthy and get your business travel done. Keeping up your workout routines while traveling has many benefits, including better sleep, better moods, and more energy.

MOVE

When you've got a day full of busy meetings ahead, make sure you have a **PFC** breakfast to fuel your body and brain.

E A T

Some days you win, some days you need to try again. Whichever kind of day it is for you, remember: it's the person who keeps getting up and trying again who wins!

RECHARGE

WWW.DAWNMCGEE.GURU

Traveling again? Yep. My #1 tip for being able to stay on plan while traveling: Ask for a fridge in your room so you can have fresh water and a shake ready to go. You can also hang on to leftovers or pick up some lighter fare for breakfast. Where there's a will, there's a way.

EAT

SEPTEMBER 17

"Strength in beauty.
Beauty in strength."

- Unknown

RECHARGE

WWW.DAWNMCGEE.GURU

Fall is in the air and it's a great time to recommit your health goals. Where do you want to be at this time next year with your health? Set (or renew) some health goals, break them down into manageable bits, and let's get started! You may want some extra support or an accountability partner to ensure you get there.

RECHARGE

When you're eating clean, it's the mindset that's most important because this is a lifestyle, not a diet.

When I go out to dinner, I plan out what I'm going to eat so that I can stay on plan.

In many restaurants, you can get a piece of naked (no salt, no butter or oil) salmon with steamed broccoli. Squeeze lemon over both for added flavor.

E A T

My son's Sensei says that "enthusiasm is caught, not taught." Attitudes are contagious. Make yours worth catching.

RECHARGE

Fall is upon us! Do you struggle with keeping up your healthy eating and workout routines this time of the year? Most of us do. Here are a few tips to keep yourself on track as the weather cools and the days get shorter:

Figure out what time of day works best for your fall schedule, and stick to it.

Start with quick cardio blasts to get the most out of even the most hurried workout.

Don't neglect your strength training workouts.

Cardio is important, and doing 30 minutes of strength training before your cardio will make it more effective.

MOVE

Do you need a helping hand to keep you on track? Join us over in my Facebook group Never Diet Again for the support, tips, and accountability you've been searching for! This is a safe space for group members to ask questions and share experiences.

*facebook.com/groups/NeverDiet

RECHARGE

Love eating eggs for the health benefits, but feeling bored of your usual veggie omelette? Try a quiche, adding egg to your favorite PFC-friendly stir-fry, or my favorite, baked egg muffin to add a little interest to your routine.

E A T

Anything worth having is worth waiting for. What goal keeps you waiting and working?

SEPTEMBER 25

How have you improved
since yesterday?

RECHARGE

WWW.DAWNMCGEE.GURU

If you want to know what could be accomplished in just 8 weeks, read what my former client Tucker Hummel had to say:

"Done with my 8-Week Challenge. Results: Lost 33 pounds, 7 inches from my waist, 4 inches from my hips, 7 inches from my chest. A special thanks to Dawn McGee for coaching me and supporting me every step of the way. Looking forward to continuing the journey from this point forward. Heck, if I can buckle down, any one of you that want to lose weight or get into a healthy way of eating surely can as well. Hit Dawn up and get involved!"

Are you ready to make a change?

RECHARGE

In the United States, obesity rates have been steadily on the rise for the past several years. Time to get off the couch and get this trend moving in the other direction!

MOVE

Let's talk about trouble spots.
Trouble spots can exist
in nutrition, in exercise, or even
just in life. What are
yours? How have you tried
to resolve them?

RECHARGE

Water sports are a great way to build extra motivation and fun into your exercise. How do you keep your workouts fresh and fun?

MOVE

As the autumn colors start to pop in New England, it's time for apple and pumpkin picking. What are your favorite fall recipes?

"We all experience challenging moments with our health and struggle with the busyness of life. The way to Get Your Body Back is 1% at a time. Imagine where you'll be 365 days from now with 1% daily progress. Make this the moment you draw your line in the sand and let your greatest health chapter begin."

- Mark Macdonald

RECHARGE

Look out! We are now entering the eating season! Do you gain weight every year at this time? It doesn't have to be the case anymore. Crush those cravings! Join the movement at Never Diet Again.

EAT

My MRFK is ready
and I'm off to pick up my kiddo.
Enjoy your travels, wherever
they may take you, and don't
forget to pack snacks!

E A T

My son and I went for a hike nearby and there were abundant climbing rocks. As he scampered around like a mountain goat, he talked about how he misses being able to climb more and how free he felt. He was so clearly in a comfortable space, happy being himself, it made me wonder how often we let ourselves get stuck in a space that isn't comfortable. This week, think of one thing that makes you feel free, and plan some time for that.

MOVE

Do you want six-pack abs?
Focus on core movements
beyond just crunches. Planks,
side planks, and a classic Pilates
set. These are all great additions
to your routine. Plus, you'll have
better posture and look leaner.

MOVE

Shout out to all you weekend warriors out there. You've been busy all week and you are going to be busy having fun all weekend. Fuel your day with a super quick and on plan breakfast. Try this egg white scramble with toasted pine nuts, garlicy spinach, and some of my favorite Benito's Hot Sauce.

E A T

Sometimes we forget that it's our differences that make the world go around, not our similarities. So many times I catch myself before I correct someone who is doing something differently than I would. And sometimes, I don't catch myself. I'm a work in progress! How about you?

RECHARGE

WWW.DAWNMCGEE.GURU

Too busy for breakfast? I almost thought the same thing this morning. And then I caught myself. Seven minutes from when I walked into my kitchen until I walked out with this great egg scramble in my hands. The key is having food in your house that you can assemble quickly - pre-packaged egg whites, avocado, tomatoes, and peppers. Enjoy!

EAT

Some days, I just have to take a deep breath and go. I'm almost always glad I did. And the stuff I was afraid of, not so scary anymore!

RECHARGE

Some days you may feel like sleeping in. Some days you may feel like you can "just wait until tomorrow's workout." Don't give in, do your workout. I'm always glad I did! I have more energy and a clearer head. What is your go-to workout when you're having a tough time getting motivated?

MOVE

Keep your head up and keep smiling. It's a beautiful day!

RECHARGE

Every day I do a little something to improve my perspective on life. It may be reading a book, charting a path to achieve my goals, or it may just be thinking about an inspiring saying. Over the years, without even realizing it, my perspective has changed. Rome wasn't built in a day, but brick by brick, one day at a time. What will you do today to improve your perspective?

RECHARGE

What kind of movement makes you happy? There isn't a one-size-fits-all workout. As long as you are moving and happy, you will find a benefit. Better mood, better food choices, better fitting clothing. It's all good, right?

MOVE

What do you have
planned for today?

RECHARGE

Spice it up! Who says breakfast has to be bland and boring? I added a little kick to my breakfast by adding some jalapenos with my sweet bell peppers. One whole egg, two egg whites, and you have a deliciously spicy alternative to the usual.

Pro tip: don't inhale too deeply when you're sauteing jalapenos!

EAT

Each new day is a new
opportunity to start again.
What will you do with your day?

RECHARGE

Think positively: You'll be happier, and who knows? Maybe things will turn out better too.

"Whether you think you can or you think you can't, you're right."

- Henry Ford

RECHARGE

Ever have a strong desire for an off plan meal, even though you just had one? Sometimes, I need to get creative to stay on plan. I love buffalo chicken pizza, but want to stay on plan. So I stir-fry chicken, one egg, tomatoes, and bell peppers, and I top it with some Frank's Hot Sauce (a bit high in sodium, but life is about compromising, right?). *phew* Cravings managed for another meal.

E A T

Wouldn't it be great to have the time for a fabulous workout every day? Some days, we can fit it in, some days we can't. Either way, don't give up. Get some movement and sweat into your days, and over time, you'll feel and see the positive results. You can do it, I know you can.

MOVE

When I got stuck inside during Hurricane Matthew, I was thankful to have a safe hotel and good food. No stress eating here! Veggie omelet and fresh fruit. Then, off to the gym! Don't workout on an empty stomach!

EAT

No time to prep! I rarely let this happen, but I just realized that lunch had to be on-the-go. I grabbed some leftover grilled chicken, avocado, and butternut squash noodles. I steamed the noodles, strained out the water, then sauteed them with the chicken and avocado. Five minutes and I'm ready to go! Thank goodness I keep a well stocked pantry and fridge! This is how your nutrition coach eats.

E A T

What does your morning routine look like? Do you start with a cup of coffee? A jog? Your morning habits set the tempo for the rest of your day. Rest, nutrition, and exercise are all important components to maintaining a youthful, healthy body! Don't skip breakfast!

RECHARGE

Do your daily habits inspire confidence? Clothing and makeup should accent a body you love, appreciate, and enjoy.

"Our food should be our medicine, and our medicine should be our food."
- Hippocrates

As we age, our bodies rely on us to provide high-quality fuel. Eating well and staying active can keep us youthful and healthy through the years. What are some foods that keep you feeling satisfied and energized?

EAT

"OMG, we have to leave for karate in 15 minutes! And we still have to get dinner ready!" This is what happened last night. Good thing we had mahi-mahi prepared. Grabbed some cashews, tomatoes, and mango to have with the fish. Ready in less than three minutes and delicious! This is how your nutrition coach goes with the flow.

EAT

Is Halloween candy your kryptonite? Do you keep eating it even after you're full? Here are three tips to survive the Halloween frenzy:

1. Eat a PFC balanced meal before your candy so you won't be hungry and craving sugar.

2. Have a few pieces. Eat them slowly and savor them.

3. If you still want something sweet, try going for a walk instead. It will give your body time to realize that it doesn't need more food.

Remember, a little chocolate won't ruin your season, but that Halloween hangover is no fun!

E A T

Focus on how to fit a workout into your busy life. Take the stairs whenever possible. Your legs will look great, and you'll get a mini mental break too!

MOVE

As the weather starts to turn to autumn, my foodie tastes turn to comfort food. Making a big pot of a yummy and healthy beef and vegetable stew fits the bill so well. You can freeze some for later and have it any day when you're stumped on what to make. Pair with a small green salad for a balanced meal.

EAT

OCTOBER 29

Sometimes it just takes a small
change to make a difference
in your life - or someone else's.

RECHARGE

WWW.DAWNMCGEE.GURU

As the fall weather encroaches, I am moving my workouts inside. Time to try some new classes at my gym! What will you do to keep your workouts fun and fresh?

MOVE

Avoid the Halloween Hangover! Help your kids learn healthy habits by pairing some fun fruit with protein and fat to help keep their blood sugar stable while they trick or treat.

E A T

Turn that frown upside down. Maximize your day by choosing to be happy! You can do it, I know you can!

RECHARGE

Sometimes I don't feel like working out, but I have a standing deal with myself to go to class, go to the gym, and if I still want to go home after 10 minutes, I can. For the past 25 years, I have not used that deal once! Sign up for some dance classes with friends and you'll have fun plus an accountability partner

MOVE

It can be a challenge to go out to eat with friends, thinking you have to choose between staying on plan and having fun, right? Not so! Try Naruto (sushi wrapped in cucumber) instead of the rice-heavy maki and you are good to go!

E A T

Sometimes, the very best you can do is just keep moving forward. Do that. And keep doing that. Eventually, you will be able to fly.

RECHARGE

Want a great rear view and great legs? Do your squats, and make sure you use proper form so you don't injure your knees or your back.

MOVE

Breakfast on my balcony, overlooking the pool. Egg white frittata with mushrooms, spinach, and fennel. I love that hotels are starting to get on board with healthier options.

EAT

Always working
on myself. You?

RECHARGE

I love these! I don't consume a lot of caffeine, but when I do, it's one of these. Delicious, natural energy sources and only 50 calories per can. Try one next time you need an afternoon pick-me-up!

mixed
berry

peach
mango

lemon
ginger

EAT

Thanksgiving is right around the corner! Set yourself up for success this holiday season. Commit to staying on plan and fitting in some extra workouts so you can splurge on your favorites.

E A T

My home away from home when I'm in Texas. It's nice to have access to a gym, but you can do a body weight workout wherever you are with just your body weight. All you need is a patch of floor and a little creativity! It'll keep you feeling healthy and young.

MOVE

New sneakers to keep me
moving comfortably!
Remember to replace yours
often. I'm grateful to
have the freedom and health
to use mine regularly.

MOVE

Some days you may be moving forward with speed and intention, some days it may be tough to move at all. As long as you keep moving towards your goals, you will get there.

RECHARGE

"Shoot for the moon. Even if you miss, you'll land among the stars."

- Les Brown

Don't be afraid to set goals.
Even if they feel ambitious,
they'll keep you on track and give
you something to work towards.
Just keep moving forward!

RECHARGE

When you dig into something that is difficult, you need to remember why you started in the first place. Why it was important to you. Recently, we built a gingerbread house with a yard, a fish pond, and a gathering of friends. I focus on my health so I can spend more time like that with my family. What is your why?

RECHARGE

We have had a lot of wild turkeys in our neighborhood. And it's so interesting to note how much slimmer they are than farm raised turkeys. Consider the parallel to humans—those of us who run and are active are leaner than people who are sedentary. So, get up and get moving if you want to be leaner! Take conference calls on a walk. Do 10 squats every hour. Do isometric core exercises while sitting at your desk. Where there is a will, there is a way - no matter how busy you are!

M O V E

Sometimes, your Plan A doesn't come to fruition. Make sure you have a Plan B and an accountability partner to support you. I'm here to help.

"Set your life on fire.
Seek those who
fan your flames."

- Rumi

If you surround yourself
with positive people who build you
up, you'll achieve so much more.

RECHARGE

We're rapidly approaching the "season of eating"! The week leading up to turkey day is a great opportunity to eat a little cleaner. You'll feel better and it'll help you stay in better control of those BLT's (bites, licks, and tastes!) that can sabotage your efforts to stay healthy.

EAT

Healthy food in an airport? You bet! Hard boiled eggs and some fresh fruit makes for a great mid-morning meal while I'm waiting for my flight.

EAT

This is my interpretation of an old tavern favorite. I skipped the fries and added fruit. Who says eating healthy is no fun?

EAT

"Make the most of yourself
by fanning the tiny, inner
sparks of possibility into
flames of achievement."

- Golda Meir

RECHARGE

Why do you want to better yourself? I do it because I want more than what I've got. I want to give back and help others. I want to be a good role model for my son. Keeping your eye on your goals and motivations keeps you moving in the right direction.

RECHARGE

What challenges are you facing in your life right now? Our challenges make us stronger, braver, smarter people.

RECHARGE

This is one of my go-to meals. It never disappoints. Mahi-mahi, grapes, and cashews. You can substitute any type of lean protein, fruit, and nuts to customize to your taste.

EAT

Looking for that extra energy without exposing your body to harmful mass-market energy drinks? Caffeine is ok for a quick boost, but instead of relying on it for your energy all the time, try clean eating—you'll be amazed at how much energy you have!

EAT

"Build a life you won't need
a vacation from."

- Unknown

This quote speaks to why I am
a nutrition coach. I am so
happy to be helping people get
healthier that I don't ever feel
like I'm just working until my
next vacation. This is my wish
for all of you as well!

RECHARGE

One of the lessons in my son's leadership class in karate: love. What a great message to teach the future leaders.

RECHARGE

It is the time of the year when we take a step back from our usual busy lives and enjoy the holidays with our loved ones. Enjoy!

RECHARGE

A long time ago, in a different life, when I was playing pool competitively, I noticed that the best players were also the luckiest. The ball rolled into the pocket when it was teetering on the edge, they usually sunk balls on the break, and so on. And then, after a while, I realized that they also worked harder than anyone else. Food for thought.

RECHARGE

The only bad workout is
the one you didn't do.

MOVE

You've heard people say that the ones who succeed simply get up one more time than they fall down? Well, let's keep on getting up! I know I will!!

RECHARGE

We're never too busy to do the stuff that's really important to us. Maybe you're not too busy to eat healthy and go to the gym. Now is always a good time to make a change.

RECHARGE

Sometimes, during this crazy holiday season, it's not the specifics of the workout that count, it's the consistency. Whether you sneak in 10 minutes of pushups, crunches, squats and jumping jack intervals, or whether you can spend time doing a longer workout, the point is JUST DO SOMETHING.

MOVE

Eat well, move daily, hydrate often, sleep lots, love your body, repeat for life.

MOVE

During this holiday season, we can easily forget about ourselves in the mad rush to do things for everyone else. Take time for yourself, cherish yourself, your beauty and your worth! If you make New Year's resolutions, make ones that let you improve 1% at a time, setting yourself up for great success!

RECHARGE

When I travel, I always hear people complain about how difficult it is to eat on plan while traveling. Let's dispel that myth. I ordered an egg white omelet with spinach, mushrooms, and tomatoes. It came with potatoes and I'll have a few of those to round out my carbs. A well balanced PFC meal. Add in hot tea, and I'm satisfied for the next few hours. What are your toughest challenges about eating on plan while traveling?

EAT

Don't let one imperfect meal ruin your day.

Looking to add some variety to your meal plan? Try a delicious and nutritious Mediterranean Quinoa Salad. It's great meatless for vegetarians, or add chicken for non-vegetarians!

E A T

"Wellness is not a medical fix, but a way of living — a lifestyle sensitive and responsive to all the dimensions of body, mind, and spirit..."

- Greg Anderson

Wellness is achieved by making permanent lifestyle changes; NOT by dieting.

RECHARGE

Remember the song, "Put one foot in front of the other, and soon you'll be walking out the door..." Every single day, every one of us makes a choice when we wake up: Get up and face the day, or pull the covers over our head and stay in bed. For some people, it's so easy and doesn't seem like a choice; we get up and get going. For some people, there are easy days and tough days. For others, it's a struggle every day. The thing is, if you keep doing the same thing, you'll get the same results. So do something different! Try something new! Be brave! I promise you'll be glad you did!

RECHARGE

Eating foods high in antioxidants will give you that extra boost naturally, so you can more easily be the superhuman you strive to be.

Not sure where to start with cleaning up your eating habits? Download my 7 Favorite Smoothie Recipes at http://bit.ly/MyFavSmoothies

EAT

What are you having for breakfast this morning?

EAT

Try keeping a food journal
for a week so you can see what
you're putting into your body.
Then work with a coach to
plan realistic changes.

EAT

Don't be tied to the scale - set non-weight related goals; for instance, training for a 5K, or learning to surf, or ski. Making your healthy living journey fun and fulfilling will keep you from losing momentum.

RECHARGE

Mondays always seem to come too soon? Be sure you're getting the necessary vitamins and minerals to keep those Monday blues away!

EAT

Figure out what your biggest obstacles are in your health journey. A busy schedule, junk food around the office, and emotional eating are all common examples of things that keep us from our weight loss goals. Do you have a community you can call on for support?

RECHARGE

Things not going as planned?
Choosing fresh fruit or a
salad as a snack helps your
body function at its best
during stressful situations.

EAT

Looking for that
mid-afternoon boost?
Here's a tip: you won't find it in
chocolate or coffee.

EAT

Holiday times can be difficult times for people for lots of reasons. Just remember this: you are good enough the way you are! Enjoy what you can and ditch the rest. And remember to breathe.

RECHARGE

This is the time of year when we have more social engagements and often de-prioritize our workouts. It's ok to have fun , but don't forget to maintain all the progress we've made this year. Enjoy your parties and your workouts this season, and you'll be proud of yourself in January!

MOVE

"Happiness is not in having what you want, but in wanting what you have."

- Rabbi Hyman Schachtel

RECHARGE

In eight days, the New Year begins. The major stigma behind resolutions is that so many people break them so quickly. I challenge you to change that.

This year, I'm resolving to build more strength. Will there be times that I want to quit? Yes. Will there be times that I feel like a failure? Probably. Will I pick myself up and try again? Definitely. Why? Because it'll be worth it.

You may have to try a lot of times to get it 'right,' but if you remember why you started in the first place, it'll keep you going.

RECHARGE

We have a fledgling tradition that our son makes us breakfast in bed during our holidays. It's such a treat and I'm so proud of him for making it a PFC meal. Lead by example and your kids will follow.

EAT

"Find joy in discovering what makes your soul happy."

- Aly Aubrey

RECHARGE

This is the best week of the year to regroup, rejuvenate and update your strategic plans for the new year. Are you ready to carry your good habits into the new year? Have you made plans to ensure your success?

RECHARGE

Exercise daily. Eat healthy.
Work hard. Stay strong.
Worry less. Dance more.
Love often. Be happy.

This is a good set of thoughts for
this time of year. Try to enjoy
some of the fun of seeing friends
and family this season instead of
getting caught up in the
commercial craziness of it all.

RECHARGE

What do you do when you get home late? Ugh. Dinner time already. Good thing we keep food in the fridge ready to get assembled. Chicken avocado salad. A great balance of protein, healthy fat, and carbs. And we avoid the fast food trap!

EAT

Snuck in a quick workout between meetings. Was it perfect? No. Was it better than sitting at my desk and waiting for the perfect time? Yep. Did I work on work stuff while on the bike? Yep. Where there is a will, there is a way.

MOVE

It's almost the last workout of the year! Did you take some time for you, to get your blood pumping? Working out always improves my mood and gives me more energy. And even if you're not at home, you can always do a couple of quick circuits: jumping jacks, squats, push-ups, plank. Rest, repeat! Your body will thank you.

MOVE

What will next year look like for you? Do you have your goals set and written down? Posted in a place where you will see them every day? Make this your best year yet! Happy New Year!

RECHARGE

NOTE ON HOLIDAYS

You may have noticed that I don't offer many tips around the subject of holidays and how to manage them. There's a good reason for that: There is no magic to managing holidays.

In a nutshell, these are the top three tips I share with clients when it comes to navigating nutrition during a holiday or special event:

1 - Decide whether you're going to be on plan or off plan.
If you're off plan, enjoy your event, don't feel guilty,
and get right back on plan next meal.

2 - If you're going to be on plan, don't go to a party/dinner hungry.
Eat at least a half a meal before you go.

3 - Minimize your alcohol intake to prevent impulse control problems.
Scope out the food options when you arrive and decide
what you're going to eat, and then stick to it.

You can get more details on my strategies for holidays, family dinners, and dining out in my Eat, Drink & Be Healthy Guide. Grab yours at
bit.ly/EatDrinkGuide.

And as always, if you have any questions, feel free to jump into my free Facebook Group, Never Diet Again. You can tag me in all your questions there!

WHAT'S NEXT?

You did it!

You made it through a whole year of finding new ways to take care of your body and bring your health to the next level. Want to keep going? Here are some options:

Visit me at my home on the web, **www.dawnmcgee.guru**

If you haven't joined my free Facebook group yet, please do! You'll find more tips and tricks there, as well as a community of like-minded people. Visit **www.facebook.com/groups/neverdiet** to check it out.

I offer a membership site where you'll have access to my entire vault of workshops, meal planning and food shopping worksheets, monthly live Q&A sessions with me, monthly sessions with other professionals including fitness trainers, time management specialists, and others, and so much more. Want more info? Visit **bit.ly/ThriveCommunityNow**

Need more simple, actionable strategies for eating well, moving, and recharging in your daily life? My program Reclaim Your Life, One Bite at a Time™ is an an intensive on making the best choices possible with consideration to your busy life. Learn more at **http://dawnmcgee.guru/services/**

Interested in working with me one-on-one? I accept a limited number of private clients each year. If you'd like to be one of them, message me at **http://dawnmcgee.guru/contact/**

Finally, if you have feedback, I'd love to hear it! I hope my books are a valuable resource for you—that can only happen if we're communicating about what you like, dislike, or need for next time.

ACKNOWLEDGEMENTS

This book would not have been possible without the help and support of so many people. First and foremost, to my family—my husband, Mike, and my son, Spencer, thank you! You are the reason why I started on my healthy living journey and why it is so important for me to be healthy—to be a good role model and to be able to be an active part of your lives.

To the team that helped this book grow from an idea to reality—Kena Roth, Cassidy Dickens, Kami Fanning, thank you for all the research, design, and support. And to the team that took the reality and brought it across the finish line—Michelle Fairbanks, Liz Thompson, and Alexa Bigwarfe, thank you for the cover, editing, and publishing; without which you would not be reading this book today.

This list wouldn't be complete without a big hug to Mark Macdonald, the Venice Nutrition coaches, and everyone who lives PFC ever 3. Meeting Mark and becoming a Venice coach was the starting point of this wonderful journey.

Almost last, but certainly not least, thank you to my friends who not only didn't laugh at me when I told them I had written a book, but who told me (without prompting) that they would most certainly buy a copy.

Finally, thank you to you, dear reader, who made a choice to start living a healthy life. Healthy living has a way of snowballing in the best possible way. The world will be a better place because of you.

HI, I'M DAWN MCGEE,
YOUR NUTRITION COACH

As a busy mom, wife, and entrepreneur, I used to struggle with my weight and get frustrated about how my clothes fit. Especially after my son was born! I was on the verge of giving up and buying bigger clothes when I got introduced to PFC (Protein, Fat, and Carbs) every 3. It gave me back control over my eating habits. I'm never starving and I lost the weight I wanted to without feeling like I was on a diet.

Now, I am passionate about helping people learn how to improve their eating habits for today and for a lifetime. As a certified and licensed Venice Nutrition coach and a long-time foodie, I focus on both the health and joy of food as fuel for your body. I want to be a driving force in bringing education on healthy eating to more people.

I want you to love your life!

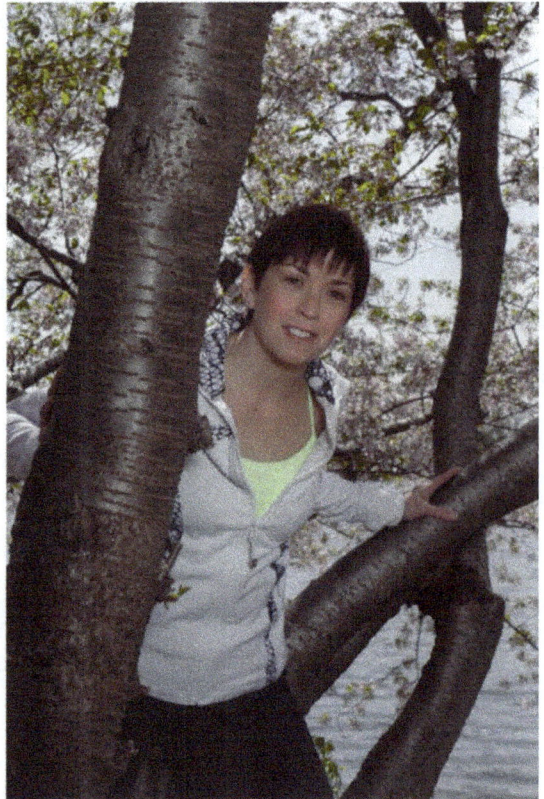

www.ingramcontent.com/pod-product-compliance
Lightning Source LLC
Chambersburg PA
CBHW080711220326
41598CB00033B/5381